INTRODUCTION

The Importance of Testosterone

Many people believe that testosterone is a hormone that only men can have. It is mainly linked to aggressiveness, muscular mass, and sexual prowess. But this strong hormone affects various aspects of physical and emotional health in both men and women, and it is essential. In women, the ovaries and adrenal glands produce smaller amounts of testosterone than in men, which is largely produced in the testes. Gaining an appreciation of the tremendous effects testosterone has on our bodies and thoughts requires an understanding of its significance.

The development of masculine traits including muscular mass, bone density, and body hair depends on testosterone. It affects fat distribution and red blood cell formation as well. In females, testosterone has a role in maintaining libido, brain function, and bone strength. Optimal testosterone levels are necessary for general health, energy, and vigor in both sexes. Many health problems, including reduced muscle mass, increased body fat, osteoporosis, and mental disorders like anxiety and depression, can be brought on by a drop in testosterone.

Beyond its physical benefits, testosterone also plays a critical role in cognitive function. It affects concentration, memory, and problem-solving abilities. Low levels of testosterone have been linked to cognitive decline and increased risk of neurodegenerative diseases such as Alzheimer's. Moreover, testosterone influences motivation, self-confidence, and emotional stability, underscoring its importance in maintaining mental health.

Why You Need to Read This Book

Many factors contribute to decreased testosterone levels in both men and women in today's fast-paced, stressful society. The modern lifestyle can be harmful to hormone health in a number of ways, including poor food choices, inactivity, exposure to environmental pollutants, and prolonged stress. Sadly, not many people are aware of these subtly harmful testosterone killers and their extensive effects.

"Worst Testosterone Killers" aims to shed light on these silent saboteurs and provide practical solutions for maintaining optimal testosterone levels. This book is not just for those experiencing symptoms of low testosterone; it is for anyone interested in improving their overall health and well-being. By understanding the various factors that impact testosterone, readers can take proactive steps to protect their hormone health and enhance their quality of life.

This book is suitable for readers with different levels of hormone knowledge since it blends scientific research with useful recommendations. This book provides insightful analysis and practical solutions for anyone interested in exercise, health, or understanding why they are not feeling as driven and energised as they once did.

How to Use This Book

"Worst Testosterone Killers" is structured to guide you through understanding testosterone, identifying factors that harm it, and implementing strategies to boost it naturally. Each chapter is designed to build on the previous one, providing a comprehensive overview of testosterone health.

The book begins with a foundational understanding of testosterone, its role in the body, and the symptoms of low testosterone. This knowledge is crucial for recognizing the importance of maintaining healthy hormone levels and understanding the impact of testosterone on various aspects of health.

The subsequent chapters explore medical conditions, psychological effects, environmental contaminants, and lifestyle choices that have a negative impact on testosterone levels. You may increase your awareness of how your daily decisions affect the health of your hormones by learning about these testosterone killers.

In the latter part of the book, you will find practical strategies to boost testosterone naturally. These include dietary recommendations, effective exercise routines, sleep optimization techniques, and stress management practices. Advanced optimization strategies and the latest research in hormone health are also discussed, providing a holistic approach to maintaining optimal testosterone levels.

Each chapter includes actionable tips and advice that you can implement immediately. Whether it's making dietary changes, incorporating new exercise routines, or adopting better sleep habits, these strategies are designed to be practical and sustainable.

The book also includes a thorough conclusion that summarizes important ideas and gives readers a plan of action. This guarantees that you may stay on course with your testosterone optimization quest and quickly access essential information.

The Journey Ahead

As you embark on this journey, remember that maintaining optimal testosterone levels is not a one-size-fits-all approach. Individual differences in genetics, lifestyle, and health status mean that what works for one person may not work for another. Therefore, it's essential to listen to your body and consult healthcare professionals when necessary.

This book aims to empower you with knowledge and tools to make informed decisions about your hormone health. By understanding the worst testosterone killers and implementing strategies to mitigate their effects, you can take control of your health and enhance your overall well-being.

So, let's begin this journey together. Turn the page and start exploring the fascinating world of testosterone, uncover the hidden killers, and discover the powerful strategies that can help you achieve optimal hormone health.

Chapter One

Understanding Testosterone

Men's testes are the main organs for producing testosterone, whereas women's ovaries and adrenal glands also produce some of it. It is essential for many body processes, such as the growth of male reproductive tissues, the maintenance of muscular mass and bone density, and the control of mood and desire. To preserve general health and wellbeing, one must comprehend the functions of testosterone as well as its significance and the variables that affect its levels.

The Role of Testosterone in the Body

1. Development and Reproductive Function:
- **Fetal Development:** Testosterone is critical during fetal development for the formation of male genitalia. The presence of the Y chromosome triggers the production of testosterone, leading to the development of male reproductive organs.

- **Puberty:** Growth of the penis and testes, deeper voice, increased muscle mass, and facial and body hair are examples of secondary sexual traits that arise from the surge in testosterone levels that occurs throughout puberty.

2. Muscle and Bone Health:

- **Muscle Mass:** Testosterone promotes protein synthesis, which is essential for muscle growth and repair. Higher testosterone levels contribute to increased muscle mass and strength.
- **Bone Density:** Testosterone lowers the incidence of osteoporosis and maintains bone density by stimulating the formation of new bone tissue. A higher risk of fractures and weaker bones can result from low testosterone levels.

3. Sexual Health and Libido:

- **Libido:** In both men and women, testosterone plays a major role in determining sexual desire. Sexual dysfunction and decreased libido can be caused by low levels.
- **Sperm Production:** In men, testosterone is necessary for the production of sperm.

Low levels can lead to decreased sperm count and fertility issues.

4. Mood and Cognitive Function:

- **Mood Regulation:** Emotional and mental health are impacted by testosterone. Low levels are associated with tiredness, irritability, and depressive symptoms.
- **Cognitive Function:** There is evidence suggesting that testosterone may play a role in cognitive functions such as memory and spatial abilities.

Factors Affecting Testosterone Levels

Changes in testosterone levels can be caused by a number of factors, including age, lifestyle, and environment. Comprehending these components can help enhance and regulate testosterone production.

1. Age:

- Testosterone levels peak during adolescence and early adulthood. After the age of 30, levels typically decline by about 1% per year. This natural decline can be influenced by lifestyle factors and overall health.

2. Lifestyle Factors:

- **Diet:** There is a strong correlation between nutrition and testosterone production. Hormone levels may suffer from a diet deficient in zinc, vitamin D, and healthy fats, among other vital minerals. Conversely, a diet rich in essential nutrients and well-balanced can support the maintenance of normal hormone levels.
- **Exercise:** Regular physical activity, particularly resistance training and high-intensity interval training (HIIT), has been shown to boost testosterone levels. Conversely, a sedentary lifestyle can lead to decreased testosterone production.
- **Sleep:** Quality sleep is crucial for testosterone production. Studies have shown that sleep deprivation can significantly lower testosterone levels.
- **Stress:** High cortisol levels from ongoing stress can prevent the body from producing testosterone. To keep testosterone levels in check, stress management practices like mindfulness, meditation, and exercise are crucial.

3. Environmental Factors:
- **Endocrine Disruptors:** Exposure to certain chemicals, known as endocrine

disruptors, can interfere with hormone production. These chemicals are found in plastics, pesticides, personal care products, and industrial pollutants.
- **Pollution:** Environmental pollutants, including heavy metals and air pollution, can negatively impact testosterone levels and overall health.

4. Health Conditions and Medications:
- A number of illnesses, including diabetes, sleep apnea, and obesity, can cause low testosterone levels. Furthermore, drugs like steroids, painkillers, and some antidepressants can prevent the body from producing testosterone.

Measuring and Diagnosing Low Testosterone

1. Symptoms of Low Testosterone:
- Typical symptoms include erectile dysfunction, fatigue, sadness, decreased libido, decreased muscular mass, and increased body fat. Since these symptoms can be mistaken for other disorders, a clinical evaluation is essential to rule out other possible causes of low testosterone.

2. Blood Tests:

- A blood test measuring total testosterone levels is typically conducted in the morning when levels are highest. Normal testosterone levels range from 300 to 1,000 ng/dL. Levels below 300 ng/dL are generally considered low.
- A more thorough understanding of hormone health may be obtained by performing further tests that measure free testosterone, luteinizing hormone (LH), and follicle-stimulating hormone (FSH).

3. Medical Evaluation:

- Conducting a thorough medical history and physical examination is necessary in order to rule out alternative causes of the symptoms. This evaluation can help determine the underlying causes of low testosterone and guide appropriate treatment.

Managing and Optimizing Testosterone Levels

1. Lifestyle Modifications:

- **Diet:** Eating a balanced diet that includes lean proteins, healthy fats, and a variety of fruits and vegetables can support testosterone production. Foods rich in zinc (e.g., oysters, red meat, poultry), vitamin D (e.g., fatty fish, fortified dairy products), and healthy fats (e.g., avocados, nuts, olive oil) are particularly beneficial.

- **Exercise:** Engaging in regular physical activity, especially resistance training and HIIT, can naturally boost testosterone levels. Incorporating compound movements like squats, deadlifts, and bench presses can be particularly effective.
- **Sleep:** To rule out other potential causes of the symptoms, a thorough medical history and physical examination are required. This assessment can guide appropriate care and help uncover the underlying causes of low testosterone.
- **Stress Management:** Implementing stress-reduction techniques such as mindfulness, meditation, deep breathing exercises, and physical activity can help lower cortisol levels and support testosterone production.

2. Supplements:
- Certain supplements have been shown to support testosterone levels. These include:
- **Zinc:** Essential for testosterone production and overall hormonal health. Supplements

can be beneficial for those with a deficiency.

- **Vitamin D:** Supports testosterone production and overall health. Supplementing can be particularly effective in persons with low levels of vitamin D.
- **Ashwagandha:** An adaptogen that can help reduce stress and improve testosterone levels.
- **Fenugreek:** Some studies suggest that fenugreek supplementation can boost testosterone levels and improve libido.

3. Medical Treatments:
- For individuals with clinically low testosterone, medical treatments may be necessary. These include:
- **Testosterone Replacement Therapy (TRT):** Involves supplementing the body with synthetic testosterone through injections, gels, patches, or pellets. TRT can effectively restore normal testosterone levels but requires regular monitoring and medical supervision.
- **Human Chorionic Gonadotropin (hCG) Therapy:** hCG stimulates the testes to produce testosterone. It is often used in

conjunction with TRT to maintain fertility and testicular size.
- **Clomiphene Citrate:** A medication that increases the body's natural testosterone production. Men who want to retain their fertility yet have low testosterone often use it off-label.

4. Advanced Techniques:

- **Red Light Therapy (RLT):** Involves exposing the body to low-level red and near-infrared light. Studies suggest it can enhance mitochondrial function, reduce inflammation, and potentially boost testosterone levels.
- **Hyperbaric Oxygen Therapy (HBOT):** Involves breathing pure oxygen in a pressurized environment. Some studies suggest potential benefits for testosterone production and overall health.

The Future of Testosterone Research

Ongoing research continues to explore the complexities of testosterone and its impact on health. Emerging areas of interest include:

1. Genetic Influences:

- Understanding the genetic factors that influence testosterone production and sensitivity can lead to more personalized approaches to hormone optimization.

2. Microbiome and Testosterone:
- Investigating the role of the gut microbiome in hormone regulation. Early research suggests that gut health may influence testosterone levels and overall hormonal balance.

3. Novel Therapies:
- Development of new therapies and interventions that can safely and effectively boost testosterone levels without adverse side effects.

For both men and women, it is critical to comprehend the vital function that testosterone plays in health. Through the identification of the factors that impact testosterone levels and the execution of tactics to enhance them, people can improve their general welfare and standard of living. The keys to sustaining good testosterone levels and enjoying the advantages of ideal hormonal health are routine monitoring, a balanced lifestyle, and well-informed decision-making. As science progresses, we will be able to successfully manage and optimize testosterone levels thanks to new discoveries and treatments.

Chapter Two

Lifestyle Factors that Kill Testosterone

Maintaining optimal testosterone levels is crucial for overall health and well-being. However, several lifestyle factors can negatively impact testosterone production, leading to a host of physical and mental health issues. This chapter delves into the key lifestyle factors that can sabotage your testosterone levels, including poor diet choices, lack of physical activity, and inadequate sleep.

Poor Diet Choices

The foods we consume play a significant role in regulating hormone levels, including testosterone. Certain dietary habits can disrupt hormone balance and lead to reduced testosterone levels.

Processed Foods

Processed foods are often high in unhealthy fats, sugars, and additives, which can negatively impact testosterone levels. These foods typically include snacks, fast food, pre-packaged meals, and sugary treats. Here's how processed foods can affect testosterone:

1. Trans Fats:
- Trans fats, commonly found in processed foods, can reduce testosterone levels and impair reproductive function. They increase inflammation and oxidative stress, which can negatively impact the testes' ability to produce testosterone.

2. High Sugar Intake:
- Excessive sugar consumption leads to spikes in insulin levels. Chronic high insulin levels can contribute to insulin resistance, which is associated with lower testosterone levels. Additionally, high sugar intake can lead to weight gain and obesity, further reducing testosterone.

3. Additives and Preservatives:
- Many processed foods contain additives and preservatives that can act as endocrine disruptors, interfering with hormone production and balance. Chemicals like bisphenol A (BPA) and phthalates, found

in some food packaging, have been linked to lower testosterone levels.

Sugar and Refined Carbohydrates

Diets high in sugar and refined carbohydrates can lead to various health issues, including decreased testosterone levels. Here's how these dietary components affect hormone health:

1. Insulin Resistance:
- High consumption of sugar and refined carbs can lead to insulin resistance, a condition where the body's cells become less responsive to insulin. Insulin resistance is associated with lower testosterone levels and can lead to type 2 diabetes, which further exacerbates hormone imbalances.

2. Weight Gain:
- Diets high in sugar and refined carbs contribute to weight gain and obesity. Excess body fat, particularly visceral fat, produces an enzyme called aromatase, which converts testosterone into estrogen, leading to reduced testosterone levels.

3. Inflammation:
- High sugar intake can increase inflammation and oxidative stress in the body. Chronic inflammation can negatively affect the Leydig cells in the testes, responsible for producing testosterone.

Alcohol and Caffeine

While moderate consumption of alcohol and caffeine is generally considered safe, excessive intake can have detrimental effects on testosterone levels.

1. Alcohol:
- Excessive alcohol consumption can impair liver function, which is crucial for hormone metabolism and detoxification. The liver converts testosterone into estrogen, and impaired liver function can lead to an imbalance, reducing testosterone levels.
- Alcohol can also increase the production of cortisol, a stress hormone that negatively impacts testosterone production. Chronic alcohol use can damage the testes, directly reducing testosterone synthesis.

2. Caffeine:

- While moderate caffeine intake can have some health benefits, excessive consumption can lead to elevated cortisol levels, which suppress testosterone production. High caffeine intake can also interfere with sleep quality, further impacting hormone balance.

Lack of Physical Activity

Regular physical activity is essential for maintaining healthy testosterone levels. Both sedentary behavior and over-training can negatively impact testosterone production.

Sedentary Lifestyle

Prolonged periods of inactivity associated with a sedentary lifestyle can result in a number of health problems, including low testosterone levels. The following are the ways that inactivity impacts hormone health:

1. Weight Gain and Obesity:

- Sedentary behavior is strongly linked to weight gain and obesity. As mentioned earlier, excess body fat can lead to increased aromatase activity, converting testosterone into estrogen and lowering testosterone levels.

2. Muscle Atrophy:
- Physical inactivity leads to muscle atrophy, or the loss of muscle mass. Since testosterone plays a critical role in muscle development, reduced muscle mass can signal the body to produce less testosterone.

3. Insulin Resistance:
- Lack of physical activity contributes to insulin resistance, which is associated with lower testosterone levels. Regular exercise improves insulin sensitivity, helping to maintain healthy hormone levels.

Over-training and Its Effects

While consistent exercise helps the body produce more testosterone, overtraining might have the opposite effect. When the body experiences excessive physical stress without sufficient recovery, overtraining takes place. This is how testosterone is affected by overtraining:

1. Elevated Cortisol Levels:

- Intense and prolonged physical activity increases cortisol levels. Chronic elevation of cortisol can suppress testosterone production, leading to hormonal imbalances.

2. Reduced Recovery:

- Over-training can lead to insufficient recovery, which is crucial for muscle repair and hormone regulation. Without adequate rest, the body's ability to produce testosterone is compromised.

3. Decreased Energy Levels:

- Over-training can lead to chronic fatigue and decreased energy levels, which can negatively impact libido and overall well-being, further contributing to reduced testosterone levels.

Inadequate Sleep

In addition to being essential to maintaining general health, sleep is also important for the creation of testosterone and other hormones. Sleep deprivation has a major effect on testosterone levels and general health.

Importance of Sleep for Hormone Regulation

1. Testosterone Production:
- Testosterone is produced during sleep, with the majority of production occurring during REM (rapid eye movement) sleep. Inadequate sleep disrupts this process, leading to reduced testosterone levels.

2. Growth Hormone Release:
- The release of growth hormone, which combines with testosterone to support muscle growth and repair, depends on sleep as well. A lack of sleep can further affect testosterone levels by interfering with the release of growth hormone.

3. Cortisol Regulation:
- Sleep helps regulate cortisol levels. Poor sleep quality or insufficient sleep can lead to elevated cortisol levels, which suppress testosterone production.

Sleep Disorders and Testosterone

Several sleep disorders can negatively impact testosterone levels, including sleep apnea and insomnia.

1. Sleep Apnea:
- Sleep apnea is a condition characterized by repeated interruptions in breathing during sleep. These interruptions can lead to reduced oxygen levels, poor sleep quality, and fragmented sleep. Studies have shown that men with sleep apnea often have lower testosterone levels.

2. Insomnia:
- Chronic sleep deprivation can result from insomnia, which is the inability to go asleep or stay asleep. Hormonal imbalances are exacerbated by chronic sleeplessness, which is linked to decreased testosterone levels and increased cortisol production.

Strategies for Mitigating Lifestyle Factors

Addressing these lifestyle factors is crucial for maintaining healthy testosterone levels. Here are some practical strategies to mitigate the impact of poor diet choices, lack of physical activity, and inadequate sleep on testosterone production.

Dietary Improvements

1. Whole Foods Diet:
- Focus on consuming a diet rich in whole foods, including fruits, vegetables, lean proteins, healthy fats, and whole grains. Whole foods provide essential nutrients that support hormone health and reduce inflammation.

2. Healthy Fats:
- Include healthy fats in your diet, such as omega-3 fatty acids found in fatty fish, flaxseeds, and walnuts. These fats are essential for hormone production and overall health.

3. Reduce Sugar and Refined Carbs:
- Limit your consumption of refined carbs and sugar. Choose complex carbs, which provide you long-lasting energy and help keep your blood sugar levels steady. Examples of these include whole grains, legumes, and veggies.

4. Moderate Alcohol and Caffeine:

- Consume alcohol and caffeine in moderation. Aim for no more than one drink per day for women and two drinks per day for men. Limit caffeine intake to 200-300 mg per day (approximately 2-3 cups of coffee).

Physical Activity

1. Regular Exercise:
- Make frequent exercise a part of your routine; this should include resistance and aerobic training. Aim for 75 minutes of vigorous-intensity aerobic activity or at least 150 minutes of moderate-intensity aerobic activity per week, in addition to two or more days of muscle-strengthening activities.

2. Balanced Training:
- Avoid over-training by balancing intense workouts with adequate rest and recovery. Listen to your body and allow sufficient time for muscle repair and regeneration.

3. Active Lifestyle:
- Reduce sedentary behavior by incorporating more physical activity into your daily routine. Take regular breaks

from sitting, walk or bike instead of driving, and engage in activities like gardening or playing sports.

Sleep Optimization

1. Sleep Hygiene:
- Establish a regular sleep routine, make your environment conducive to rest, and refrain from using electronics and caffeine right before bed to practice good sleep hygiene.

2. Address Sleep Disorders:
- If you suspect you have a sleep disorder such as sleep apnea or insomnia, seek medical evaluation and treatment. Continuous positive airway pressure (CPAP) therapy can help manage sleep apnea, while cognitive-behavioral therapy for insomnia (CBT-I) can improve sleep quality.

3. Stress Management:
- Manage stress through relaxation techniques such as meditation, deep breathing exercises, yoga, and mindfulness. Reducing stress can help

improve sleep quality and support healthy testosterone levels.

Chapter Three

Environmental Testosterone Killers

While lifestyle factors like diet, exercise, and sleep have a significant impact on testosterone levels, environmental factors also play a crucial role. Various environmental toxins and pollutants can disrupt hormone balance and negatively affect testosterone production. This chapter explores the primary environmental testosterone killers, including endocrine-disrupting chemicals (EDCs), heavy metals, and pollutants, and offers practical strategies to mitigate their impact.

Endocrine-Disrupting Chemicals (EDCs)

Endocrine-disrupting chemicals (EDCs) are substances that can interfere with the body's hormonal system. They are found in many everyday products and can have significant negative effects on testosterone levels.

Bisphenol A (BPA)

Bisphenol A (BPA) is a chemical commonly used in the production of polycarbonate plastics and epoxy resins. It is found in a variety of consumer goods, including food and beverage containers, thermal paper receipts, and dental sealants.

1. Sources of BPA Exposure:

- **Food Containers:** BPA is used in the lining of canned foods and in plastic containers that may leach BPA into food and beverages, especially when heated.
- **Receipts:** Thermal paper receipts contain BPA, which can be absorbed through the skin upon handling.
- Household Items: BPA is found in a variety of plastic products, such as water bottles, kitchen utensils, and storage containers.

2. Impact on Testosterone:

- BPA can mimic the structure and function of estrogen, binding to estrogen receptors and disrupting the hormonal balance.
- Research has indicated that exposure to BPA can cause a decrease in testosterone levels by disrupting the Leydig cells in the testes, which are in charge of producing testosterone.

3. Mitigation Strategies:

- **Avoid Plastics:** Use glass, stainless steel, or BPA-free plastic containers for food and beverages.
- **Limit Canned Foods:** Reduce consumption of canned foods and opt for fresh or frozen alternatives.
- **Handle Receipts Sparingly:** Minimize contact with thermal paper receipts and wash hands after handling them.

Phthalates

Phthalates are a group of chemicals used to make plastics more flexible and durable. They are commonly found in a wide range of products, including personal care items, household goods, and medical devices.

1. Sources of Phthalate Exposure:

Personal Care Products: Phthalates are used in fragrances, lotions, shampoos, and cosmetics.

Plastics: They are found in vinyl flooring, shower curtains, and plastic packaging.

Medical Devices: Some medical devices, such as IV bags and tubing, contain phthalates.

2. Impact on Testosterone:

- Phthalates are known to interfere with the endocrine system by disrupting the production and function of testosterone.
- Phthalate exposure has been connected to decreased testosterone levels, worse sperm quality, and problems with male child development.

3. Mitigation Strategies:

- **Choose Phthalate-Free Products:** Opt for personal care products labeled as phthalate-free.
- **Reduce Plastic Use:** Use glass, metal, or phthalate-free polymers as substitutes for plastic products.
- **Ventilate Your Home:** Ensure proper ventilation to reduce indoor air pollution from phthalates in household items.

Pesticides and Herbicides

The hormone balance and testosterone levels can be affected by chemicals found in pesticides and herbicides used in agriculture. These chemicals act as endocrine disruptors.

1. Sources of Exposure:

- **Food:** Residues of pesticides and herbicides can be found on conventionally grown fruits and vegetables.
- **Water:** Runoff from agricultural fields can contaminate water supplies with pesticide residues.
- **Occupational Exposure:** Individuals working in agriculture or landscaping may have direct exposure to these chemicals.

2. Impact on Testosterone:
- Many pesticides and herbicides can mimic or block hormones, disrupting the endocrine system and reducing testosterone levels.
- Numerous pesticides, including organochlorines and organophosphates, have been linked in studies to decreased testosterone levels and problems with reproduction.

3. Mitigation Strategies:
- **Eat Organic:** Choose organic produce to reduce exposure to pesticide residues.
- **Wash Produce:** Thoroughly wash fruits and vegetables to remove surface pesticides.

- **Filter Water:** Use water filters that can remove pesticide residues from drinking water.

Heavy Metals

Heavy metals, such as lead, mercury, and cadmium, are environmental pollutants that can have serious health effects, including disruption of hormone balance and reduction of testosterone levels.

Lead

Lead is a toxic metal found in various environmental sources, including old paint, contaminated soil, and industrial emissions.

1. Sources of Lead Exposure:
- **Old Paint:** Lead-based paints were commonly used in homes built before 1978.
- **Contaminated Soil:** Lead can persist in soil near industrial sites and urban areas.
- **Drinking Water:** Lead pipes and plumbing fixtures can leach lead into drinking water.

2. Impact on Testosterone:

- Lead exposure can impair the function of the testes, reducing testosterone production.
- Studies have shown that elevated lead levels in the blood are associated with lower testosterone levels and decreased sperm quality.

3. Mitigation Strategies:
- **Test for Lead:** Have your home tested for lead if it was built before 1978.
- **Avoid Contaminated Areas:** Limit exposure to contaminated soil, particularly for children.

Filter Water: Use water filters certified to remove lead.

Mercury

Mercury is a toxic metal found in certain types of fish, industrial emissions, and dental amalgams.

1. Sources of Mercury Exposure:
- **Fish:** Large predatory fish, such as shark, swordfish, and king mackerel, can contain high levels of mercury.

- **Industrial Emissions:** Coal-fired power plants and certain industrial processes release mercury into the air and water.
- **Dental Amalgams:** Mercury is used in some dental fillings.

2. Impact on Testosterone:

- Exposure to mercury can cause endocrine system disruption, which lowers testosterone levels and affects reproductive function.
- Studies have shown that mercury can interfere with the function of the hypothalamic-pituitary-gonadal (HPG) axis, which regulates testosterone production.

3. Mitigation Strategies:

- **Limit Fish Consumption:** Avoid or limit consumption of high-mercury fish and choose low-mercury options such as salmon, sardines, and trout.
- **Choose Alternatives:** If you have dental amalgams, discuss alternatives with your dentist.
- **Reduce Industrial Exposure:** Avoid areas with high levels of industrial pollution and advocate for cleaner energy sources.

Cadmium

Cadmium is a toxic metal found in tobacco smoke, certain foods, and industrial emissions.

1. Sources of Cadmium Exposure:
- **Tobacco Smoke:** Smoking is a major source of cadmium exposure.
- **Food:** Certain foods, such as shellfish, organ meats, and leafy vegetables, can contain cadmium.
- **Industrial Emissions:** Cadmium is released into the environment through mining, smelting, and manufacturing processes.

2. Impact on Testosterone:
- Cadmium exposure can damage the testes, reducing testosterone production and sperm quality.
- Studies have shown that cadmium can interfere with the function of Leydig cells, which are responsible for producing testosterone.

3. Mitigation Strategies:
- **Quit Smoking:** Avoid tobacco smoke to reduce cadmium exposure.

- **Monitor Food Sources:** Be mindful of cadmium levels in foods and opt for lower-cadmium options.
- **Reduce Industrial Exposure:** Limit exposure to industrial emissions and advocate for stricter environmental regulations.

Air and Water Pollutants

Air and water pollutants, including industrial chemicals and vehicle emissions, can have significant effects on hormone balance and testosterone levels.

Air Pollution

Air pollution, particularly in urban and industrial areas, contains a mix of harmful substances that can disrupt hormonal balance.

1. Sources of Air Pollution:
- **Vehicle Emissions:** Combustion engines release pollutants such as nitrogen oxides, sulfur dioxide, and particulate matter.
- **Industrial Emissions:** Factories and power plants emit various pollutants, including heavy metals, volatile organic

compounds (VOCs), and polycyclic aromatic hydrocarbons (PAHs).
- **Household Pollutants:** Indoor air can be contaminated by chemicals from cleaning products, building materials, and tobacco smoke.

2. Impact on Testosterone:
- Reproductive dysfunction and lower testosterone levels have been related to exposure to air pollution.
- Pollutants such as PAHs and heavy metals can interfere with the endocrine system, reducing testosterone production and increasing oxidative stress.

3. Mitigation Strategies:
- **Reduce Exposure:** Limit outdoor activities on days with high air pollution levels and use air purifiers indoors.
- **Ventilate Your Home:** Ensure proper ventilation to reduce indoor air pollution.
- **Support Clean Energy:** Advocate for policies that reduce air pollution from vehicles and industrial sources.

Water Pollution

Water contaminants, such as medicines, industrial pollutants, and agricultural waste, can alter the balance of hormones and lower testosterone levels.

1. Sources of Water Pollution:
- **Industrial Discharges:** Factories and power plants can release pollutants into water bodies.
- **Agricultural Runoff:** Pesticides, herbicides, and fertilizers from agricultural fields can contaminate water supplies.
- **Pharmaceuticals:** Medications and personal care products can enter water systems through improper disposal and sewage.

2. Impact on Testosterone:
- Water contaminants such as heavy metals, endocrine disruptors, and pharmaceuticals can interfere with hormone production and regulation.
- Studies have shown that exposure to contaminated water can lead to reduced testosterone levels and reproductive

Chapter Four

Psychological Factors Affecting Testosterone

Psychological issues also affect testosterone levels in addition to environmental influences and physical health. The synthesis and regulation of testosterone can be profoundly impacted by stress, anxiety, depression, and other mental health conditions. This chapter explores the numerous psychological factors that impact testosterone levels and offers solutions to lessen their detrimental effects.

Stress and Its Impact on Testosterone

Stress is a natural response to challenging situations, but chronic stress can have detrimental effects on hormonal balance, including testosterone levels.

The Stress Response and Hormones

When the body perceives a threat, it activates the stress response, releasing hormones such as cortisol and adrenaline. This response is designed to prepare the body for immediate action, commonly known as the "fight-or-flight" response.

1. Cortisol Production:

- Cortisol, a glucocorticoid hormone produced by the adrenal glands, plays a crucial role in managing stress. While essential for survival, chronic elevation of cortisol levels can have negative health effects.
- High cortisol levels suppress the hypothalamic-pituitary-gonadal (HPG) axis, which regulates testosterone production. Prolonged stress can lead to reduced testosterone levels as the body prioritizes cortisol production over reproductive hormones.

2. Adrenaline Release:

- Adrenaline, also known as epinephrine, is another hormone released during the stress response. It increases heart rate, blood pressure, and energy availability. While beneficial in acute stress situations, chronic activation can strain the body and affect hormone balance.

Chronic Stress and Testosterone

Chronic stress, characterized by prolonged or recurrent stressors, can significantly impact testosterone levels and overall health.

1. Psychological Stress:
- Mental stressors, such as work-related pressures, financial worries, and relationship issues, can lead to chronic stress. Psychological stress is a major factor in reducing testosterone levels.
- Studies have shown that individuals experiencing chronic psychological stress have lower testosterone levels compared to those with lower stress levels.

2. Physical Stress:
- Physical stressors, such as illness, injury, and over-training, can also contribute to chronic stress. Physical stress impacts the body's ability to produce testosterone by increasing cortisol levels and suppressing the HPG axis.
- Overtraining syndrome, which is typified by chronic fatigue, decreased performance, and hormonal imbalances, including low testosterone levels, can result from overtraining, especially in sports.

Mitigation Strategies for Stress

Managing stress is crucial for maintaining healthy testosterone levels. Here are some effective strategies to reduce stress and support hormone balance:

1. Mindfulness and Meditation:
- Reducing stress and cortisol levels can be achieved through mindfulness and meditation practices. Relaxation and mental health can be enhanced by methods including progressive muscle relaxation, guided graphical representation, and deep breathing.
- Regular meditation has been shown to reduce stress, improve mood, and support healthy hormone levels, including testosterone.

2. Exercise:
- Regular physical activity is a powerful stress reliever. Exercise promotes the release of endorphins, which are natural mood enhancers, and helps reduce cortisol levels.
- Engaging in activities such as yoga, tai chi, or moderate aerobic exercise can be

particularly effective in managing stress
and supporting hormonal balance.

3. Healthy Lifestyle:
- Maintaining a healthy lifestyle, including
a balanced diet, adequate sleep, and social
support, can help mitigate the effects of
stress on testosterone levels.
- Prioritizing sleep and practicing good
sleep hygiene can improve resilience to
stress and support overall hormonal health.

4. Counseling and Therapy:
- Seeking professional assistance in the
form of counseling or therapy can be quite
beneficial in helping one manage ongoing
stress. Cognitive-behavioral therapy (CBT)
can help enhance coping strategies and is
especially useful in treating anxiety and
stress.

Anxiety and Its Effects on Testosterone

Anxiety, characterized by excessive worry
and fear, can also negatively impact
testosterone levels. Like stress, chronic
anxiety can lead to hormonal imbalances and
reduced testosterone production.

Anxiety and Hormone Regulation

Anxiety triggers the release of stress hormones, including cortisol, which can disrupt the balance of reproductive hormones.

1. Cortisol and Testosterone:
- Chronic anxiety leads to elevated cortisol levels, which suppress testosterone production. High cortisol levels interfere with the function of the HPG axis and reduce the body's ability to produce and maintain adequate testosterone levels.
- Studies have shown that individuals with chronic anxiety disorders often have lower testosterone levels compared to those without anxiety.

2. Psychological Impact:
- Anxiety can have an impact on one's mental health and general wellbeing, resulting in symptoms including fatigue, irritability, and diminished libido. Low testosterone levels are linked to these symptoms as well, which feeds a vicious cycle in which worry makes hormone imbalances worse.

Mitigation Strategies for Anxiety

Managing anxiety is essential for maintaining healthy testosterone levels and overall well-being. Here are some strategies to reduce anxiety and support hormonal balance:

1. Therapeutic Interventions:
- Cognitive-behavioral therapy (CBT) is an effective treatment for anxiety. CBT helps individuals identify and challenge negative thought patterns and develop coping strategies to manage anxiety.
- Other therapeutic approaches, such as acceptance and commitment therapy (ACT) and mindfulness-based stress reduction (MBSR), can also be beneficial in reducing anxiety and improving mental health.

2. Medication:
- In some cases, medication may be necessary to manage anxiety. Selective serotonin reuptake inhibitors (SSRIs) and benzodiazepines are commonly prescribed to reduce anxiety symptoms.
- It is important to consult with a healthcare professional to determine the most appropriate treatment for anxiety.

3. Lifestyle Modifications:

- Maintaining a healthy lifestyle can assist with hormone balance and anxiety management. Anxiety management requires a balanced diet, regular exercise, and enough sleep.
- Reducing caffeine and alcohol intake, which can exacerbate anxiety symptoms, is also important.

4. Relaxation Techniques:

- Anxiety can be controlled by incorporating relaxation techniques into everyday activities. Relaxation techniques that help lower anxiety levels include yoga, meditation, deep breathing exercises, and progressive muscle relaxation.

Depression and Its Impact on Testosterone

A frequent mental health condition called depression is characterized by enduring melancholy, hopelessness, and disinterest in activities. Both total health and testosterone levels can be greatly impacted by depression.

Depression and Hormonal Imbalances

Depression is associated with hormonal imbalances, including reduced testosterone levels. The relationship between depression and testosterone is bidirectional, meaning that low testosterone can contribute to depression, and depression can lead to lower testosterone levels.

1. Hypothalamic-Pituitary-Adrenal (HPA) Axis:
- Depression affects the HPA axis, which regulates stress response and hormone production. Dysregulation of the HPA axis can lead to elevated cortisol levels and reduced testosterone production.
- Studies have shown that individuals with depression often have lower testosterone levels compared to those without depression.

2. Inflammation:
- Elevations of inflammation in the body are linked to depression. Prolonged inflammation can lower testosterone levels and impede the generation of hormones.
- Inflammatory markers, such as C-reactive protein (CRP) and interleukin-6 (IL-6), are often elevated in individuals with

depression and are associated with lower testosterone levels.

Mitigation Strategies for Depression

Addressing depression is crucial for maintaining healthy testosterone levels and overall well-being. Here are some strategies to manage depression and support hormone balance:

1. Therapeutic Interventions:
- Psychotherapy, particularly cognitive-behavioral therapy (CBT), is an effective treatment for depression. CBT helps individuals identify and challenge negative thought patterns and develop coping strategies to manage depression.
- Other therapeutic approaches, such as interpersonal therapy (IPT) and dialectical behavior therapy (DBT), can also be beneficial in treating depression.

2. Medication:
- Antidepressant medications, such as selective serotonin reuptake inhibitors (SSRIs) and serotonin-norepinephrine reuptake inhibitors (SNRIs), are commonly prescribed to treat depression.

- It is important to work with a healthcare professional to determine the most appropriate treatment for depression and to monitor for any potential side effects on hormone levels.

3. Lifestyle Modifications:
- Adopting a healthy lifestyle can help manage depression and support hormone balance. Regular exercise, a balanced diet, and adequate sleep are crucial components of depression management.
- Depression symptoms can also be lessened by partaking in socially supportive activities, such as going out with loved ones and taking part in community events.

4. Complementary Therapies:
- Complementary therapies, such as acupuncture, massage therapy, and herbal supplements, can also be beneficial in managing depression and supporting overall health.
- Mindfulness-based practices, such as meditation and yoga, can help reduce depression symptoms and promote relaxation.

Social Isolation and Its Effects on Testosterone

Social isolation, or the lack of social connections and interactions, can negatively impact mental health and testosterone levels.

The Importance of Social Connections

Humans are social beings, and social connections play a crucial role in mental and physical health. Social interactions stimulate the release of hormones that promote well-being, including oxytocin and serotonin.

1. Hormonal Effects of Social Isolation:
- Social isolation can lead to increased levels of stress and anxiety, which can negatively impact testosterone levels. The absence of social support can exacerbate feelings of loneliness and depression, further reducing testosterone production.
- According to studies, those who are socially connected have higher testosterone levels and generally better health than people who are socially disconnected.

2. Mental Health Impact:

- Social isolation is associated with increased risk of mental health disorders, such as depression and anxiety, which can negatively impact hormone balance.
- The lack of social interaction can lead to feelings of loneliness, low self-esteem, and reduced motivation, all of which can contribute to lower testosterone levels

Chapter Five

Medical Conditions and Medications

Medication side effects and other medical issues can have a substantial impact on testosterone levels. The subject matter here explores the effects of various illnesses, conditions, and therapies on the synthesis and control of testosterone. Effective management of testosterone levels can be achieved by being aware of these impacts.

Medical Conditions Impacting Testosterone

Several medical conditions can directly or indirectly affect testosterone levels. These conditions may interfere with hormone production, regulation, or function.

Hypogonadism

Hypogonadism is a condition characterized by low testosterone levels due to the testes' inability to produce sufficient hormones or issues with the hypothalamic-pituitary axis.

1. Primary Hypogonadism:

- **Causes:** The cause of primary hypogonadism is an issue with the testes. Hemochromatosis, testicular damage, mumps orchitis, Klinefelter syndrome, and undescended testicles are among the common causes.
- **Impact:** In primary hypogonadism, the testes fail to produce adequate testosterone despite normal or elevated levels of luteinizing hormone (LH) and follicle-stimulating hormone (FSH).

2. Secondary Hypogonadism:

- **Causes:** Issues with the hypothalamus or pituitary gland, which control the production of testosterone, might result in secondary hypogonadism. Pituitary problems, tumors, Kallmann syndrome, obesity, and long-term illnesses are among the causes.
- **Impact:** In secondary hypogonadism, low levels of LH and FSH lead to insufficient stimulation of the testes, resulting in low testosterone levels.

3. Symptoms and Diagnosis:

- **Symptoms:** Low libido, erectile dysfunction, reduced muscle mass, fatigue, depression, and infertility.
- **Diagnosis:** Blood tests to measure testosterone levels, LH, FSH, and other relevant hormones. Imaging studies and genetic tests may be required for further evaluation.

4. Treatment:
- Testosterone replacement therapy (TRT) is the primary treatment for hypogonadism. It can be administered via injections, gels, patches, or implants.
- Addressing underlying causes, such as weight loss in obesity or treating pituitary disorders, is also crucial.

Metabolic Syndrome and Diabetes

Metabolic syndrome and diabetes are associated with insulin resistance and obesity, which can negatively impact testosterone levels.

1. Metabolic Syndrome:
- **Components:** Metabolic syndrome includes central obesity, hypertension, dyslipidemia, and insulin resistance.

- **Impact on Testosterone:** Elevated levels of aromatase, an enzyme that changes testosterone into estrogen, can result from insulin resistance and obesity, which lowers the amount of accessible testosterone. Reduced testosterone is also a result of inflammation and elevated cortisol levels.

2. Diabetes:

- **Type 2 Diabetes:** Type 2 diabetes is often associated with obesity and insulin resistance, both of which can lower testosterone levels.
- **Impact on Testosterone:** Chronic hyperglycemia and insulin resistance can impair Leydig cell function in the testes, reducing testosterone production.

3. Symptoms and Diagnosis:

- **Symptoms:** Low testosterone in metabolic syndrome and diabetes can cause erectile dysfunction, fatigue, decreased libido, and loss of muscle mass.
- **Diagnosis:** Blood tests to measure fasting glucose, HbA1c, lipid profile, and testosterone levels.

4. Treatment:

- **Lifestyle Changes:** Weight loss, diet modification, and regular exercise can improve insulin sensitivity and help restore testosterone levels.
- **Medications:** Diabetes medications like metformin have been shown to enhance insulin resistance and may have a beneficial effect on testosterone levels. For people with verified low testosterone, TRT may be taken into consideration.

Obesity

Obesity is a significant risk factor for low testosterone levels due to increased aromatase activity and hormonal imbalances.

1. Impact on Testosterone:
- **Aromatase Activity:** Fat tissue contains aromatase, which converts testosterone to estrogen, leading to lower testosterone levels.
- **Inflammation:** Obesity is associated with chronic low-grade inflammation, which can negatively affect testosterone production.

2. Symptoms and Diagnosis:

- **Symptoms:** Fatigue, reduced libido, erectile dysfunction, and decreased muscle mass.
- **Diagnosis:** measurements of waist circumference, testosterone levels in the blood, and body mass index (BMI).

3. Treatment:
- **Weight Loss:** Dietary changes, physical activity, and behavioral therapy to promote weight loss and reduce fat tissue.
- **Surgical Options:** Bariatric surgery for severe obesity can significantly improve hormonal balance and testosterone levels.
- **TRT:** Testosterone replacement therapy may be considered for obese individuals with clinically low testosterone levels.

Sleep Apnea

Sleep apnea is a sleep disorder characterized by repeated interruptions in breathing during sleep, which can negatively affect testosterone levels.

1. Impact on Testosterone:
- **Hypoxia:** Repeated episodes of hypoxia (low oxygen levels) during sleep can impair testosterone production.

- **Sleep Disruption:** Poor sleep quality and fragmented sleep can disrupt the normal diurnal rhythm of testosterone secretion.

2. Symptoms and Diagnosis:

- **Symptoms:** Daytime fatigue, loud snoring, gasping for air during sleep, reduced libido, and erectile dysfunction.
- **Diagnosis:** Sleep studies (polysomnography) to diagnose sleep apnea and blood tests to measure testosterone levels.

3. Treatment:

- **Continuous Positive Airway Pressure (CPAP):** CPAP therapy is the standard treatment for obstructive sleep apnea and can improve sleep quality and testosterone levels.
- **Lifestyle Changes:** Weight loss, avoiding alcohol and sedatives, and sleeping on one's side can help reduce sleep apnea severity.
- **TRT:** Testosterone replacement therapy may be considered for individuals with low testosterone levels secondary to sleep apnea.

Medications Impacting Testosterone

Some drugs may affect the synthesis, function, or control of testosterone. It is essential to comprehend the possible adverse reactions of these drugs in order to control testosterone levels.

Opioids

Opioids are powerful pain-relieving medications that can negatively affect testosterone levels, especially with long-term use.

1. Mechanism of Impact:
- **Hypothalamic Suppression:** Opioids can suppress the hypothalamic-pituitary-gonadal (HPG) axis, reducing the release of gonadotropin-releasing hormone (GnRH) and subsequently lowering testosterone production.
- **Direct Effects:** Opioids may also have direct effects on the testes, impairing testosterone production.

2. Symptoms and Diagnosis:
- **Symptoms:** Fatigue, reduced libido, erectile dysfunction, and decreased muscle mass.

- **Diagnosis:** Blood tests to measure testosterone levels and review of medication history.

3. Management:

- **Dose Adjustment:** Elevating testosterone levels can be achieved by lowering the dosage of opioids or by using non-opioid pain management techniques.
- **TRT:** Testosterone replacement therapy may be considered for individuals with opioid-induced hypogonadism.

Glucocorticoids

Anti-inflammatory drugs called glucocorticoids, including prednisone, are frequently prescribed to treat a range of inflammatory and autoimmune diseases. Testosterone levels may be impacted by prolonged use.

1. Mechanism of Impact:

- **HPG Axis Suppression:** Glucocorticoids can suppress the HPG axis, reducing the release of LH and FSH, leading to lower testosterone production.

- **Cortisol Effects:** Elevated cortisol levels due to glucocorticoid use can negatively impact testosterone production.

2. Symptoms and Diagnosis:
- **Symptoms:** Fatigue, reduced libido, erectile dysfunction, and decreased muscle mass.
- **Diagnosis:** Measuring testosterone levels through blood tests and reviewing past drug usage.

3. Management:
- **Dose Adjustment:** Reducing the dose of glucocorticoids or switching to alternative treatments with less impact on the HPG axis can help improve testosterone levels.
- **TRT:** Testosterone replacement therapy may be considered for individuals with glucocorticoid-induced hypogonadism.

Antidepressants

Certain antidepressants, particularly selective serotonin reuptake inhibitors (SSRIs), can affect testosterone levels and sexual function.

1. Mechanism of Impact:

- **Serotonin Regulation:** SSRIs increase serotonin levels, which can inhibit sexual arousal and testosterone production.
- **Hormonal Imbalance:** Antidepressants can disrupt the balance of neurotransmitters and hormones, impacting testosterone levels.

2. Symptoms and Diagnosis:
- **Symptoms:** Reduced libido, erectile dysfunction, and decreased sexual satisfaction.
- **Diagnosis:** Review of medication history and evaluation of symptoms.

3. Management:
- **Medication Adjustment:** Switching the class of antidepressants to one with less sexual adverse effects or lowering the dosage can help enhance sexual function and testosterone levels.
- **Combination Therapy:** Adding medications to counteract sexual side effects, such as bupropion, can also be beneficial.

Anti-Androgens and Hormonal Therapies

Medications used to treat prostate cancer, such as anti-androgens and androgen deprivation therapy (ADT), can significantly reduce testosterone levels.

1. Mechanism of Impact:
- **Androgen Blockade:** Anti-androgens block the action of testosterone on its receptors, reducing its effects.
- **Hormonal Suppression:** ADT reduces testosterone production by inhibiting the release of GnRH, LH, and FSH.

2. Symptoms and Diagnosis:
- **Symptoms:** Fatigue, reduced libido, erectile dysfunction, decreased muscle mass, and hot flashes.
- **Diagnosis:** Blood tests to measure testosterone levels and review of treatment history.

3. Management:
- **Alternative Treatments:** Exploring alternative treatments for prostate cancer that have less impact on testosterone levels.
- **Supportive Therapies:** Engaging in lifestyle modifications, physical therapy, and psychological support to manage

symptoms associated with low testosterone levels.

Chapter Six

Age and Testosterone

Testosterone, a key hormone in males, plays a vital role in various bodily functions, including muscle mass, bone density, red blood cell production, mood regulation, and sexual health. As men age, testosterone levels naturally decline, impacting these functions. Understanding the relationship between age and testosterone is essential for addressing age-related health concerns.

Testosterone Levels Across the Lifespan

Testosterone levels vary significantly throughout a man's life. They peak during adolescence and early adulthood, then gradually decline with age.

Adolescence and Early Adulthood

1. Puberty:
- **Hormonal Surge:** During puberty, testosterone levels rise sharply, triggering the development of secondary sexual

characteristics such as increased muscle mass, deepening of the voice, and growth of facial and body hair.
- **Peak Levels:** Testosterone levels peak in late teens to early twenties, with normal ranges typically between 300 to 1,000 ng/dL (nanograms per deciliter).

2. Early Adulthood:
- **Stability:** Testosterone levels remain relatively stable through the twenties and early thirties, supporting physical and reproductive health.

Midlife Decline

1. Gradual Decline:
- **Age-Related Decrease:** Testosterone levels begin to decline at a rate of about 1-2% per year after the age of 30. By age 40, levels may decrease by approximately 20% from their peak.
- **Impact on Health:** This decline can contribute to various health issues, including reduced muscle mass, increased body fat, decreased libido, and mood changes.

2. Andropause:

- **Concept:** Andropause, sometimes referred to as male menopause, describes the period of life when men experience a significant drop in testosterone levels. This typically occurs in men aged 40 to 55.
- **Symptoms:** Common symptoms include fatigue, depression, irritability, reduced libido, erectile dysfunction, and loss of muscle mass and strength.

Older Age

1. Continued Decline:

- **Advanced Age:** Testosterone levels continue to decline into older age. By age 70, testosterone levels may be about half of what they were at peak levels.
- **Health Implications:** Low testosterone in older men is associated with increased risk of osteoporosis, frailty, cognitive decline, and metabolic syndrome.

2. Variability:

- **Individual Differences:** The rate of decline and the impact on health vary widely among individuals. Some men maintain relatively high levels of testosterone into old age, while others experience more rapid declines.

Causes of Age-Related Testosterone Decline

Several factors contribute to the decline in testosterone levels with age, including changes in the hypothalamic-pituitary-gonadal (HPG) axis, lifestyle factors, and comorbid medical conditions.

Hypothalamic-Pituitary-Gonadal Axis

1. HPG Axis Regulation:
- **Normal Function:** The HPG axis regulates testosterone production through a feedback loop involving the hypothalamus, pituitary gland, and testes.
- **Age-Related Changes:** Aging affects the sensitivity and function of this axis. The hypothalamus and pituitary gland produce less gonadotropin-releasing hormone (GnRH) and luteinizing hormone (LH), respectively, leading to reduced stimulation of the testes.

2. Leydig Cell Function:
- **Reduced Efficiency:** Leydig cells in the testes, responsible for testosterone production, become less efficient with age.

This decline in function contributes significantly to lower testosterone levels.

Lifestyle Factors

1. Obesity:
- **Impact on Hormones:** Increased body fat, particularly visceral fat, leads to higher levels of aromatase, an enzyme that converts testosterone to estrogen, thus lowering testosterone levels.
- **Metabolic Syndrome:** Obesity is often associated with metabolic syndrome, which further exacerbates hormonal imbalances.

2. Physical Activity:
- **Exercise and Testosterone:** Regular physical activity, especially resistance training, helps maintain higher testosterone levels. Sedentary lifestyles contribute to a more rapid decline in testosterone.

3. Diet and Nutrition:
- **Nutritional Deficiencies:** Poor diet and nutritional deficiencies can impact testosterone production. Adequate intake of zinc, vitamin D, and healthy fats is

essential for maintaining testosterone levels.

4. Alcohol and Smoking:

Substance Abuse: Excessive alcohol consumption and smoking can negatively affect testosterone levels and overall health.

Medical Conditions

1. Chronic Diseases:

- **Diabetes and Cardiovascular Disease:** Conditions like type 2 diabetes and cardiovascular disease are associated with lower testosterone levels due to their impact on overall health and hormone regulation.
- **Obstructive Sleep Apnea:** Sleep disorders, particularly obstructive sleep apnea, are linked to reduced testosterone levels.

2. Medications:

- **Impact of Drugs:** Certain medications, such as opioids, glucocorticoids, and antidepressants, can lower testosterone levels by affecting hormone production and regulation.

Symptoms of Low Testosterone

Recognizing the symptoms of low testosterone is crucial for early intervention and management. Symptoms can be physical, emotional, and cognitive.

Physical Symptoms

1. Decreased Muscle Mass and Strength:
- **Muscle Atrophy:** Lower testosterone levels lead to a reduction in muscle protein synthesis, resulting in muscle atrophy and decreased strength.
- **Exercise Tolerance:** Reduced testosterone can impact exercise tolerance and recovery.

2. Increased Body Fat:
- **Fat Distribution:** Men with low testosterone often experience increased body fat, particularly around the abdomen, due to hormonal imbalances and decreased metabolic rate.

3. Bone Density:
Osteoporosis Risk: Low testosterone is associated with decreased bone density and increased risk of osteoporosis and fractures.

4. Sexual Health:

- **Libido and Erectile Function:** Reduced libido and erectile dysfunction are common symptoms of low testosterone. These issues can significantly impact quality of life and relationships.

Emotional and Cognitive Symptoms

1. Mood Changes:

- **Depression and Irritability:** Low testosterone is linked to mood disorders, including depression and irritability. Hormonal changes can affect neurotransmitter levels, impacting mood regulation.

2. Cognitive Function:

- **Memory and Concentration:** Testosterone plays a role in cognitive function. Lower levels are associated with difficulties in memory, concentration, and cognitive performance.

Diagnosis and Treatment of Low Testosterone

Proper diagnosis and treatment of low testosterone are essential for managing symptoms and improving quality of life.

Diagnosis

1. Blood Tests:
- **Testosterone Levels:** Total testosterone levels are typically measured in the morning when levels are highest. A level below 300 ng/dL is generally considered low.
- **Additional Tests:** Free testosterone, LH, FSH, and other hormone levels may be evaluated to determine the underlying cause.

2. Symptom Assessment:
- **Clinical Evaluation:** A thorough assessment of symptoms and medical history is crucial for diagnosis. Questionnaires and symptom checklists can help quantify the impact of low testosterone.

Treatment Options

1. Testosterone Replacement Therapy (TRT):

- **Forms of TRT:** TRT can be administered via injections, gels, patches, or implants. The choice of method depends on individual preference and medical considerations.
- **Benefits and Risks:** TRT can alleviate symptoms of low testosterone, improve muscle mass and strength, enhance libido, and improve mood. However, it carries risks, including potential cardiovascular issues, prostate health concerns, and erythrocytosis.

2. Lifestyle Modifications:

- **Diet and Exercise:** Maintaining a healthy diet rich in essential nutrients and engaging in regular physical activity can help support testosterone levels.
- **Weight Management:** Achieving and maintaining a healthy weight is crucial for hormonal balance.

3. Managing Underlying Conditions:

- **Chronic Disease Management:** Addressing underlying medical conditions, such as diabetes and sleep apnea, can improve testosterone levels and overall health.

- **Medication Review:** Evaluating and adjusting medications that may impact testosterone levels is important.

4. Alternative Therapies:
- **Herbal Supplements:** Some herbal supplements, such as ashwagandha and fenugreek, have shown potential in supporting testosterone levels. However, their efficacy and safety require further research.

5. Psychological Support:
- **Counseling and Therapy:** Addressing emotional and cognitive symptoms through counseling and therapy can improve overall well-being and quality of life.

Addressing age-related health issues requires an understanding of the link between age and testosterone. Men's naturally declining testosterone levels as they age affect several body systems. The effects of aging on testosterone levels can be controlled by identifying the signs of low testosterone, comprehending the contributing causes, and investigating therapy alternatives. Men can age well and retain better health by taking a

comprehensive strategy that combines
medical care, lifestyle changes, and
psychological support.

Chapter Seven

Strategies to Boost Testosterone Naturally

Men's health is greatly influenced by testosterone, which has an impact on everything from mood and desire to muscle mass and bone density. Although testosterone levels normally decrease as people age, there are a number of natural remedies and lifestyle modifications that can help keep or even raise testosterone levels. The evidence-based strategies to increase testosterone production naturally are covered in this chapter.

1. Healthy Diet
A diet high in vital nutrients and well-balanced can have a big impact on testosterone levels. For the purpose of sustaining and increasing testosterone, some meals and nutrients are especially advantageous.

a. Macronutrients Balance
1. Proteins:

- **Importance:** Protein is essential for muscle repair and growth, which indirectly supports testosterone levels.
- **Sources:** Include lean meats, fish, eggs, dairy products, legumes, and nuts in your diet.

2. Fats:

- **Healthy Fats:** Healthy fats are critical for testosterone production.
- **Sources:** Incorporate sources of unsaturated fats such as avocados, nuts, seeds, and olive oil. Omega-3 fatty acids found in fatty fish like salmon and flaxseeds are particularly beneficial.

3. Carbohydrates:

- **Energy:** Carbohydrates are crucial for energy, especially during intense exercise.
- **Sources:** Opt for complex carbohydrates such as whole grains, fruits, and vegetables.

b. Micronutrients

1. Zinc:

- **Role:** Zinc is vital for testosterone production and the functioning of the reproductive system.
- **Sources:** Oysters, beef, spinach, pumpkin seeds, and lentils are excellent sources of zinc.

2. Vitamin D:

- **Role:** Vitamin D plays a role in hormone production and maintaining healthy testosterone levels.
- **Sources:** Sunlight exposure is the best source. Additionally, fatty fish, fortified dairy products, and egg yolks can help.

3. Magnesium:

- Role: Magnesium supports muscle function and overall hormonal balance.
- **Sources:** Green leafy vegetables, nuts, seeds, and whole grains are rich in magnesium.

4. Vitamin B:

- **Role:** B vitamins, especially B6, play a role in testosterone production.

- **Sources:** Chicken, fish, potatoes, bananas, and fortified cereals.

c. Avoid Processed Foods and Sugar

1. Impact on Testosterone: Excessive sugar and processed food intake can lead to insulin resistance and weight gain, which negatively affects testosterone levels.

2. Healthy Alternatives: Opt for whole, unprocessed foods, and reduce intake of sugary drinks and snacks.

3. Regular Exercise

One of the most natural ways to raise testosterone levels is through regular exercise, especially strength training.

a. Resistance Training

1. Impact on Testosterone:

- **Mechanism:** Resistance training, such as weightlifting, stimulates muscle growth, which in turn can boost testosterone production.
- **Exercise Examples:** Squats, deadlifts, bench presses, and other compound movements are particularly effective.

2. Frequency and Intensity:

- **Guidelines:** Engage in resistance training exercises 3-4 times a week, focusing on different muscle groups.
- **Intensity:** Use weights that challenge you but still allow for proper form to maximize benefits and minimize injury risk.

b. High-Intensity Interval Training (HIIT)

1. Impact on Testosterone:

- **Mechanism:** HIIT workouts, which involve short bursts of intense activity followed by rest or low-intensity exercise, can also boost testosterone levels.
- **Exercise Examples:** Sprints, cycling, and bodyweight exercises like burpees and jump squats.

2. Frequency and Duration:

- **Guidelines:** Incorporate HIIT sessions 1-2 times per week, with each session lasting around 20-30 minutes.

c. Consistency

- **Long-Term Benefits:** Consistency in exercise routines is key to maintaining healthy testosterone levels.
- **Variety:** Mix different types of exercises to prevent boredom and maintain overall fitness.

4. Adequate Sleep

Quality sleep is crucial for maintaining optimal testosterone levels.

a. Sleep Duration

1. Recommended Amount: Aim for 7-9 hours of sleep per night.
Impact on Hormones: Inadequate sleep can disrupt the circadian rhythm and reduce testosterone production.

b. Sleep Quality

1. Environment: Create a sleep-friendly environment by keeping your bedroom cool, dark, and quiet.
2. Routine: Establish a consistent sleep schedule by going to bed and waking up at the same time every day.

c. Avoid Sleep Disruptors

1. Electronics: Try to avoid using screens right before bed as blue light might disrupt the body's melatonin production.
2. Caffeine and Alcohol: Avoid consuming caffeine and alcohol close to bedtime, as they can disrupt sleep patterns.

4. Stress Management

Chronic stress can lead to elevated cortisol levels, which negatively affect testosterone.

a. Relaxation Techniques

1. Meditation and Mindfulness: Practices such as meditation and mindfulness can reduce stress and lower cortisol levels.
2. Deep Breathing: Deep breathing exercises can help manage stress and promote relaxation.

b. Physical Activity

1. Exercise Benefits: Regular exercise is not only good for physical health but also for reducing stress levels.

2. Nature Walks: Spending time in nature can have a calming effect and help reduce stress.

c. Time Management

1. Prioritizing Tasks: Efficient time management can reduce stress by helping you prioritize tasks and avoid feeling overwhelmed.
2. Breaks: Take regular breaks during work to avoid burnout and maintain mental health.

5. Maintaining a Healthy Weight

Achieving and maintaining a healthy weight is crucial for optimal testosterone levels.

a. Impact of Obesity

1. Hormonal Imbalance: Excess body fat, particularly visceral fat, increases aromatase activity, which converts testosterone to estrogen.
2. Insulin Resistance: Obesity is often linked with insulin resistance, which can negatively impact testosterone levels.

b. Weight Loss Strategies

1. Diet and Exercise: Combining a healthy diet with regular exercise is the most effective way to lose weight.

2. Consistency: Sustainable weight loss requires consistent lifestyle changes rather than temporary diets.

c. Monitoring Progress

1. Regular Check-Ins: Regularly monitor your weight and body composition to track progress.

2. Adjustments: Make necessary adjustments to your diet and exercise routine based on your progress.

6. Limiting Alcohol and Avoiding Smoking

Both alcohol and smoking can negatively impact testosterone levels.

a. Alcohol

1. Moderation: Limit alcohol consumption to moderate levels, defined as up to two drinks per day for men.

2. Impact on Hormones: Excessive alcohol intake can disrupt the endocrine system and reduce testosterone levels.

b. Smoking

1. Quitting: Smoking cessation is crucial for improving overall health and maintaining healthy testosterone levels.
2. Support: Seek support through counseling, nicotine replacement therapy, or support groups to quit smoking.

7. Herbal Supplements

Certain herbal supplements have demonstrated the ability to boost testosterone levels. But it's crucial to proceed cautiously and get advice from a medical professional.

a. Ashwagandha

1. Benefits: Ashwagandha is an adaptogen that can help reduce stress and increase testosterone levels.
2. Research: Studies suggest that ashwagandha supplementation can lead to significant increases in testosterone levels in stressed individuals.

b. Fenugreek

1. Benefits: Fenugreek may support testosterone levels by inhibiting enzymes that convert testosterone to estrogen.

2. Research: Some studies have shown that fenugreek supplementation can improve testosterone levels and sexual function.

c. D-Aspartic Acid

1. Benefits: D-Aspartic acid is an amino acid that may boost testosterone levels by increasing luteinizing hormone (LH) production.

2. Research: Some evidence suggests that D-Aspartic acid can increase testosterone levels in men with low baseline levels.

8. Regular Health Check-Ups

It is essential to have regular checkups to track testosterone levels and general wellness.

a. Blood Tests

Testosterone Levels: Regular blood tests to measure total and free testosterone levels can help track changes over time.

Other Hormones: Monitoring other hormones such as LH, FSH, and cortisol is also important.

b. Addressing Medical Conditions

Underlying Conditions: Managing chronic conditions such as diabetes, hypertension, and sleep apnea can positively impact testosterone levels.
Medication Review: Regularly review medications with your healthcare provider to identify any that may impact testosterone levels.

Conclusion

Testosterone is a vital hormone that affects a variety of aspects of a man's health and wellbeing, such as his ability to perform physically, mentally, and sexually. We've looked at a number of variables that can lower testosterone levels throughout this book and provided solutions to lessen their effects. Our extensive range of topics covers medical conditions, the effects of aging, and advanced strategies for optimization, in addition to the fundamentals of testosterone and how lifestyle, environment, and psychology affect its production. All of these topics are designed to help you maintain and increase your testosterone levels in a healthy and natural way.

Summary of Key Points

1. Understanding Testosterone:
- Testosterone is essential for muscle growth, bone density, and overall vitality. It plays a significant role in male reproductive health and secondary sexual characteristics.

- Recognizing the signs of low testosterone, such as fatigue, depression, and reduced libido, is crucial for early intervention and treatment.

2. Lifestyle Factors that Kill Testosterone:

- Poor diet, lack of exercise, insufficient sleep, and chronic stress are major lifestyle factors that can lower testosterone levels.
- Simple changes such as adopting a balanced diet, engaging in regular physical activity, prioritizing sleep, and managing stress can significantly improve testosterone levels.

3. Environmental Testosterone Killers:

- Exposure to endocrine-disrupting chemicals (EDCs) found in plastics, pesticides, and personal care products can negatively affect hormone production.
- Reducing exposure by choosing organic foods, using glass containers, and selecting natural personal care products can help protect testosterone levels.

4. Psychological Factors Affecting Testosterone:

- Chronic stress, anxiety, and depression can lead to elevated cortisol levels, which inhibit testosterone production.
- Implementing stress-reduction techniques such as mindfulness, meditation, and physical exercise can enhance mental health and support hormonal balance.

5. Medical Conditions and Medications:

- Conditions like obesity, diabetes, and sleep apnea can significantly impact testosterone levels. Certain medications can also interfere with hormone production.
- Managing underlying health conditions and reviewing medications with a healthcare provider are essential steps in maintaining optimal testosterone levels.

6. Age and Testosterone:

- Testosterone levels naturally decline with age, but lifestyle interventions can slow this decline.
- Engaging in resistance training, maintaining a healthy diet, and staying active are key strategies for older adults to sustain testosterone levels.

7. Strategies to Boost Testosterone Naturally:

- A combination of healthy eating, regular exercise, adequate sleep, and stress management forms the foundation for naturally boosting testosterone.
- Specific foods rich in zinc, vitamin D, and healthy fats can support testosterone production.

8. Advanced Testosterone Optimization:

- For those seeking further enhancement, advanced strategies such as hormonal therapies (TRT, hCG therapy, clomiphene citrate), cutting-edge supplements (boron, shilajit, mucuna pruriens), and biohacking techniques (red light therapy, hyperbaric oxygen therapy) can be considered.
- These advanced methods should be pursued under medical supervision to ensure safety and efficacy.

The Path Forward

Maintaining optimal testosterone levels is a dynamic process that involves continuous effort and adaptation. The key to success lies in a holistic approach that integrates multiple facets of lifestyle and health management.

Here are some actionable steps to help you on your journey:

1. Regular Monitoring:
- Regular blood tests to monitor testosterone and other related hormones can help track progress and identify issues early. Working with a healthcare provider to interpret these results is crucial.

2. Personalized Approach:
- Since every person is different, what works for one may not work for another. Adapting your strategy to your goals, lifestyle, and current state of health is crucial for successful testosterone optimization.

3. Consistency and Patience:
- Changes in testosterone levels and overall health take time. Consistency in implementing lifestyle changes and patience in seeing results are key to long-term success.

4. Professional Guidance:
- Consulting with healthcare providers, including endocrinologists, nutritionists, and fitness experts, can provide valuable

insights and personalized recommendations.

5. Continuous Learning:

- Making smarter selections can be facilitated by keeping up with the most recent findings and developments in hormone health research. It can be helpful to participate in health forums, go to seminars, and subscribe to reliable health journals.

The Bigger Picture

While optimizing testosterone levels is important for enhancing various aspects of health, it is equally crucial to focus on overall well-being. A holistic approach that balances physical, mental, and emotional health will yield the best results. Here are some broader considerations:

1. Mental and Emotional Health:

- Cultivating strong relationships, engaging in fulfilling activities, and seeking professional help when needed can support mental and emotional health, which in turn positively impacts hormonal balance.

2. Healthy Habits:

- Developing and maintaining healthy habits, such as regular physical activity, balanced nutrition, and sufficient sleep, contribute to overall well-being and support optimal testosterone levels.

3. Sustainable Practices:

- You and the community can safeguard hormonal health by incorporating sustainable activities into your daily life, such as lowering your exposure to environmental contaminants, buying eco-friendly products, and pushing for healthier living conditions.

4. Preventive Health Care:

- Regular check-ups, preventive screenings, and proactive management of health conditions can prevent many issues that negatively impact testosterone levels and overall health.

Final Thoughts

The natural and efficient optimization of testosterone levels is a complex process that calls for a dedication to healthy living and lifelong learning. Through comprehension of the factors that impact testosterone and application of the tactics outlined in this book, you can proactively strive towards augmenting your hormonal balance and general welfare.

Remember that health is a journey, not a destination. Stay informed, stay motivated, and prioritize your well-being. With the right knowledge and approach, you can achieve and maintain optimal testosterone levels, leading to a healthier, more vibrant life.

To sum up, there is more to the quest of ideal testosterone levels than just the hormone. It's about adopting a way of living that promotes general health, vitality, and wellbeing. You may maximize the benefits of balanced hormones and increase your testosterone levels by making educated decisions and adopting proactive measures. Cheers to your well-being and prosperity on the journey!